HEALTHCARE TEAMS

Building Continuous Quality Improvement

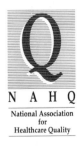

Facilitator's Guide

PETER MEARS

Department of Management
University of Louisville
Louisville, Kentucky

Q
N A H Q
National Association
for
Healthcare Quality

S^{t}L

St. Lucie Press

Phone: (407) 274-9906
Fax: (407) 274-9927

S$_L^t$

Published by
St. Lucie Press
100 E. Linton Blvd., Suite 403B
Delray Beach, FL 33483

Preface

This facilitator's guide is a companion to *Healthcare Teams: Building Continuous Quality Improvement.* This guide provides:

- Lesson plans including suggested time allocation

- Masters that can be used to create your own transparencies

- Quality bucks photocopy masters

- A method for randomly assigning participants to teams

- A "little instructor" who will offer suggestions and share ideas

Always read what the little instructor has to say about a chapter. The little instructor will share potential problems with you so that you will know what to expect (i.e., watch out for) in the chapter.

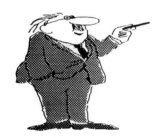

The little instructor is offering this advice for your consideration because we've been there; we know that the instructor is "under the gun" and needs someone on his or her side.

You will have to "break the mold" in these team-building sessions. The typical healthcare participant has been trained to operate as an individual: to be a go-getter, a self-starter, and to work individually. Even if assigned to teams, people do not view one another as resources. In fact, the prevailing tendency is to view one another as competitors. About the only thing your employees hold in common with each other is that they all receive paychecks from the same organization. That is, they have been trained in how to function effectively as members of a team.

Our objective in these team-building sessions is to help build organizational teams that will serve as the basis for empowered teams. Team participants will rotate team positions, and team members will critically evaluate the interactions which occurred at the end of each exercise. By doing this, we are creating an environment in which participants can learn how to learn.

Contents

Appendices

Introduction

Facilitator's Role

A facilitator/instructor can assist participants in learning how to function effectively in teams. Simply performing the chapter exercises is not enough: teams must learn how to evaluate the interactions that occurred in reaching a decision and then refine their interaction skills the next time they perform an exercise. That is, we are teaching the team members how to improve themselves by the process of "learning how to learn."

What You Will Need

- Participants: management and key staff

- Scheduled times: schedule well in advance

- Meeting room: off-site is preferred

- An overhead projector and screen, if you are going to use the transparencies

- Blackboard and chalk, or a large flip-chart and felt-tip pens

- Copies of the companion book, *Healthcare Teams: Building Continuous Quality Improvement* (one copy per participant)

- Lesson plans (see next topic)

If possible, limit the number of participants in a training session to 25 (or so) for maximum group interactions. Participants will be grouped into teams of five or six for breakout sessions. These teams will then report back to the larger group for discussions.

You will have to develop and distribute dates and times for the training series well in advance. Schedule at least one room and, if possible, an adjacent breakout room. This team development program fits nicely into an extended $1\frac{1}{2}$-hour lunch period. Eleven meetings will be required to cover all the topics. Do **not** schedule lengthy meetings or allow the meetings to expand to consume unrealistic amounts of time.

Interruptions for which participants must leave to handle "emergency" problems are disruptive and should be avoided. As a facilitator, you must frankly address this problem with the group.

Lesson Plans

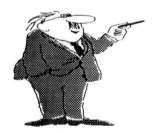

Lesson plans are needed to add focus to your meetings. It is all too easy to get together for pleasant discussions about team building without accomplishing anything. Read ahead, and use the transparency masters to create your own transparencies, which can be used to guide discussions.

Lesson plans are provided for eleven $1\frac{1}{2}$-hour individual sessions. Another approach is to combine the sessions in a two-day retreat.

Topics and Time Allocations (1½-Hour Periods)

Meeting	Chapter/Topic/Exercise	Little Instructor's Suggestions
1	**Chapter 1: Teamwork and Synergy** Exercise 1: Knowing Your Team Members	Use general transparencies. Let teams "run over" on Exercise 1.
2	**Chapter 2: Contributors to CQI** Deming's Guide Exercise 2: Deming's Audit Crosby's Guide	Transparencies entitled "Your Analysis" can be used to encourage participants to analyze group processes.
3	**Chapter 2: Contributors to CQI (continued)** Exercise 3: Crosby's Audit Juran's Guide Exercise 4: Juran's Audit	Exercise 3 (Crosby's Audit) is relatively simple. Limit discussion time. You might complete this ahead of schedule. If so, discuss Exercise 10 on team rules that will be required of all teams.
4	**Chapter 3: Empowerment** Exercise 5: What Is Empowerment? Exercise 6: Team Process Control Exercise 7: Measuring Medical Quality	There won't be enough time to complete Exercise 7. You might want to come back to this later.
5	**Chapter 4: Supportive Team Cultures** Team-Player Styles Sample Team Rules Reaching a Consensus Exercise 8: And In This Corner... Exercise 9: Admissions Problem	Exercise 6 on process control is very useful. If time permits, ask participants to repeat the process by selecting a second application.
6	**Chapter 5: Team-Building Phases** Exercise 10: Written Team Rules Exercise 11: Team Assessment Exercise 12: General Peer Feedback Exercise 13: Detailed Peer Evaluation Exercise 14: Self-Assessment	Do not allocate class time to Exercise 10. Have teams be ready to turn in team rules when you reach this session. Devote most of the time to evaluations. Remind the participants to be open-minded and to use this feedback as an educational opportunity.

Topics and Time Allocations (1½-Hour Periods) (continued)

Meeting	Chapter/Topic/Exercise	Little Instructor's Suggestions
7	**Chapter 6: Understanding How We Think** Developing Trust Colored Hat Thinking Exercise 15: Norm Violation Exercise 16: Pardon Me, Doctor, But... Exercise 17: The Room Is Not Clean?	If you cannot provide colored hats, use colored pieces of paper. Ask participants to pick up the appropriate color before making a comment. This is a powerful learning experience. Share the observers' reports among groups.
8	**Chapter 7: Member Service Roles** Exercise 18: Declining Patients Exercise 19: Why Can't You Return My Phone Calls Exercise 20: My Son, The Future Doctor	Select two or three of the exercises. After the teams analyze their observers' reports, ask observers to discuss their general findings. (Participant names are only mentioned within the team.)
9	**Chapter 8: Expanded Team Member Roles** Group Task Functions Exercise 21: Please Answer the Phone Exercise 22: No, We Can't Improve Our Services Exercise 23: Pill Pusher Blues Exercise 24: Maintenance, When?	Select two of the exercises. The objective at this point is to develop a basis where the team can learn how to learn. Be sure to schedule sufficient time for the team to discuss the observer's report.
10	**Chapter 9: Expanding Team Skills** Exercise 25: Nurse, I'm Hungry Exercise 26: Staff Problems Exercise 27: Where Do I Park?	Select two or three exercises.
11	**Chapter 9: Expanding Team Skills (continued)** Exercise 28: Insurance Hassles Exercise 29: Now What? Exercise 30: Team Assessment **Chapter 10: Teams, Teams, and More Teams**	Try random team assignments (see appendix) to see if consensus can be reached with different team members. Use transparencies to guide the discussion on how to apply teams within an organization.

Quality Bucks

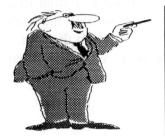

Quality bucks are not only fun, but they also serve as an important reinforcement to participants: their quality ideas make a difference. Furthermore, if you can arrange to have an auction at the end of the sessions, where anyone can bid on inexpensive memorabilia using their quality bucks, you will drive home an important point. The participants who learned how to work together as a team will develop clever and innovative bidding schemes and acquire the majority of the items.

Full-size copies of the quality bucks are provided in Appendix A in denominations of 50, 100, and 200. The 50 buck is shown here.

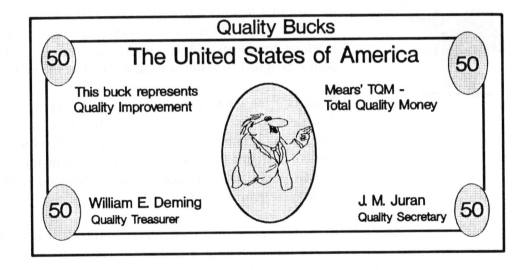

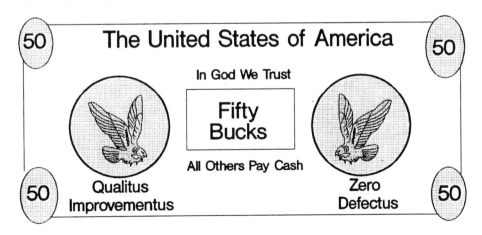

The quality bucks are near normal size and, if photocopied on green paper and trimmed, are attractive and, to say the least, novel. If you do not have access to a copier that can copy a two-sided original to a single-sided copy, it probably isn't worth the effort to copy the back side of the quality bucks. Just copy the front side, and trim the copies slightly outside of the border line. (See Appendix A for additional ideas.)

Team Assignments

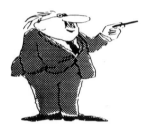

I normally allow participants to select whichever team they want, but the size of a team is restricted to from four to six participants (never less than four). However, in order to give everyone experience in reaching consensus with varying team members, participants are randomly assigned to teams toward the end of the course.

A method for randomly assigning participants to teams is shown in Appendix B. Assign a number to each student on the class roll. The first student is numbered 1, the second 2, and so forth. Then locate the random assignment table that corresponds to the number of teams desired, and read off the name that corresponds to the number in the random assignment table.

If you have a group of participants who have a social interest in being on the same team, they will not concentrate on building their team interaction skills. Randomly assign the participants to teams at the first session.

Chapter 1

Teamwork and Synergy

Objective	To explain the concept of teams, assign students to teams, and get students to appreciate the diversity and knowledge of the various team members
Pages	Pages 1–14 in *Healthcare Teams: Building Continuous Quality Improvement*
Exercises	1 Knowing Your Team Members
Transparencies	1-1 Advantages of Teamwork
	1-2 Major Elements of Synergy
	1-3 Characteristics of an Effective Team (Part 1)
	1-4 Characteristics of an Effective Team (Part 2)
	1-5 What Have I Gotten Into?

After assigning each participant to a team, use the transparencies you created from the transparency masters to guide the review of the quality contributors. Let the teams "run over" on Exercise 1, but afterward remind them to gauge their completion time better.

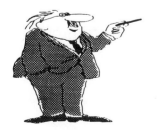

Advantages of Teamwork

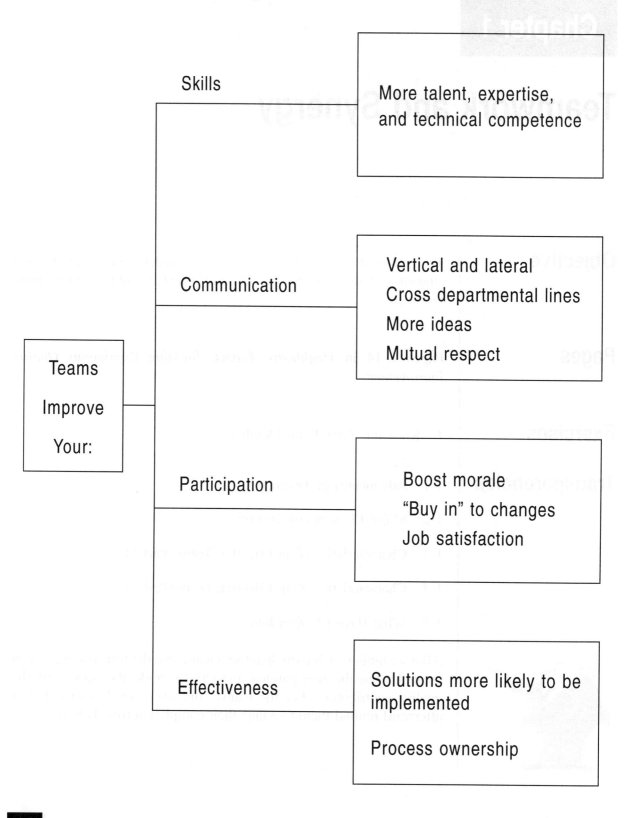

Teams Improve Your:

Skills — More talent, expertise, and technical competence

Communication
- Vertical and lateral
- Cross departmental lines
- More ideas
- Mutual respect

Participation
- Boost morale
- "Buy in" to changes
- Job satisfaction

Effectiveness
- Solutions more likely to be implemented
- Process ownership

Major Elements of Synergy

- **Listening and clarifying**
  Concentrate on what is being said

- **Supporting**
  Create a positive climate

- **Quality**
  Make a personal commitment to improve

- **Acceptance**
  Respect other members' viewpoints

- **Feedback**
  Honest communication

Characteristics of an Effective Team (Part 1)

- ■ The atmosphere is informal and relaxed, without obvious tension.

- ■ There is much discussion in which everyone participates.
  Discussion is focused.

- ■ The team's task is understood and accepted by the members.

- ■ Members listen to each other!
  Every idea is given a hearing.

- ■ The team is comfortable with disagreement and does not avoid conflict simply to keep everything in agreement.

Characteristics of an Effective Team
(Part 2)

■ Decisions are reached by a consensus.

■ Criticism is frequent, frank, and relatively comfortable.
There are no personal attacks.

■ People are free to express their feelings and ideas on the team's problems.

■ When action is taken, clear assignments are made and accepted.

■ The leader does not dominate, nor does the team.

■ The team is self-conscious about how it functions and examines how it is performing.

What Have I Gotten Into?

■ **Forming**

Stage where the team is first formed.

■ **Storming**

Stage where impatience with progress occurs.

■ **Norming**

Team members start to help one another out.

■ **Performing**

Stage where the mature team understands its strengths and weaknesses.
Members are satisfied with progress.

Chapter 2

Contributors to Continuous Quality Improvement

Objective	To begin the process of working as a team, while applying the thinking of the quality leaders to practical problems
Pages	Pages 15–60 in *Healthcare Teams: Building Continuous Quality Improvement*
Exercises	2 Deming's Audit
	3 Crosby's Audit
	4 Juran's Audit
Transparencies	2-1 Continuous Quality Improvement
	2-2 Continuous Quality Improvement Overview
	2-3 Deming's Guide to Quality (Part 1)
	2-4 Deming's Guide to Quality (Part 2)
	2-5 Deming's Audit: Assigned Teams (for Exercise 2)
	2-6 Exercise 2: Your Analysis
	2-7 Crosby: Hangings Will Continue

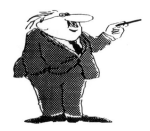

After assigning each participant to a team, use the transparencies you created from the transparency masters as a guide to reviewing the quality contributors.

These initial exercises are designed so that team members can get to know one another before concentrating on more advanced team-building skills. Participants are learning how to work together in teams while learning about quality concepts.

Do not allow the teams to get bogged down in excessive detail. Stress that Dr. Deming strongly believes that management owns the process and must find any problems with it (point 5) and then take action to eliminate variance. Encourage the team to evaluate Juran's thinking. Would most U.S. hospital administrators be more likely to accept Deming's thinking or Juran's thinking?

The answer, of course, is that Juran's thinking is far easier for managers to accept because of the accounting-type reporting format. Adoption of Dr. Deming's philosophy requires a fundamental change in the way business is conducted, and many administrators are reluctant to give up their control of the process.

The following transparencies can be used to ensure that participants are paying attention to the group processes:

2-6   Exercise 2: Your Analysis
        Did everyone participate?

2-10   Exercise 3: Your Analysis
        Change your behavior.

2-16   Exercise 4: Your Analysis
        Encourage the group to work together.
        Anyone may be asked to give the team report.

Continuous Quality Improvement

IS	IS NOT
A cultural change	An overnight cure
Responsibility of top management	Delegated to subordinates
A systematic way to improve services	A new program
A structured approach to solving problems	"Fighting fire"
Conveyed by action	Conveyed by slogans
Practiced by everyone	A specialist discipline
Team involved	A "Lone Ranger" activity

Continuous Quality Improvement (CQI)

■ Overview

    ■ Deming

        ■ Crosby

            ■ Juran

                ■ Malcolm Baldrige
                   National Quality Award

Concepts flow from Deming

CQI is...

Continuous improvement in satisfying customers

Reducing the variation in products or services

Deming's Guide to Quality (Part 1)

Types of Quality: Quality of design

Quality of conformance

Quality of performance

Deming's 14 Points:

1 Constancy toward improvement

Mission statement

2 New philosophy: No longer tolerate mistakes or delays

Quality is defined as surpassing customer needs

3 Cease dependence on mass inspection

Inspection does not make goods/services better

4 End practice of awarding based on price

Measure quality along with price

5 Find problems

Eliminate all variation: special vs. common

6 Train people

Identify goals and train to meet goals

Deming's Guide to Quality (Part 2)

7 Use modern supervision

Get rid of performance appraisals

8 Drive out fear

Working climate is very important

9 Break down barriers between departments

10 Eliminate numerical goals

Get rid of management by objectives

11 Eliminate numerical work standards

Quotas don't separate common and special variation

12 Remove barriers that rob pride of workmanship

13 Program of education and training

14 Push program for never-ending improvement

Deming's Audit

Break into your assigned teams.

Then select a healthcare organization, and using Deming's principles as a guide:

■   Identify three of their strongest points

■   Identify three of their weakest points

Why?

Be creative in your analysis.

Exercise 2: Your Analysis

To learn how to function effectively as a team:

- Start becoming aware of the group dynamics

- Think in terms of changing your behavior

- Each member must actively contribute

- Each member must move the conversation forward

- The leader must attempt to balance the opportunity to contribute

So,

- Did everyone participate?

- Did everyone participate equally?

- Could a general agreement be reached through discussion?

For the next exercise:

- Be more aware of the group processes

CQI Contributor:
Crosby

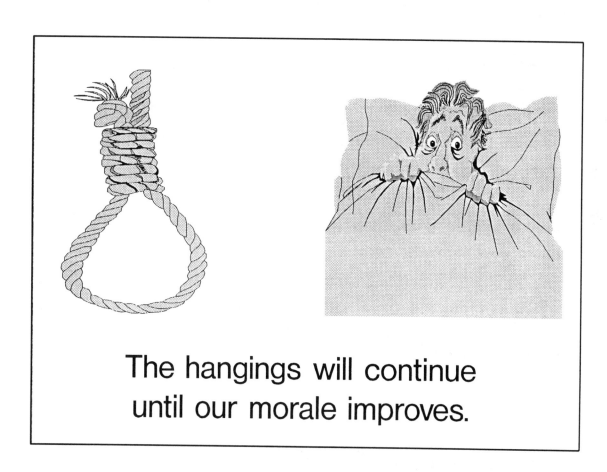

The hangings will continue
until our morale improves.

Crosby takes a humanistic approach
to improving quality

Crosby:
Quality without Tears

Hassled people do not produce quality work

You do **NOT** want a program to eliminate hassle

Eating a sandwich is a program; raising children is a process—You are never done with a process

Definition of quality: **DIRFT**
(Do It Right the First Time!)

Look at process and identify opportunities for errors

The performance standard is zero errors

We tend to accept errors as a way of doing business

Very high hidden cost

Crosby's Audit

Break into your assigned teams.

Then select a healthcare organization, and using Crosby's principles as a guide:

■ Identify three of their strongest points

■ Identify three of their weakest points

Why?

Be creative in your analysis.

Exercise 3: Your Analysis

To learn how to function effectively as a team:

■ You **MUST** change **YOUR** behavior

■ Each member must move the conversation forward

■ All members should contribute equally

■ Each member should think in terms of how he or she contributed to the group, not what was said

■ Role of team leader must be rotated for each exercise so that everyone obtains experience—no exceptions

When trying to reach a general agreement in a group:

■ Concentrate on the issues, and do not introduce personalities into the discussion

■ Do **NOT** vote on issues.

Try to reach a general agreement that the group can live with

For the next exercise:

■ Practice positive reinforcement

Juran:
Leadership for Quality

No one is against quality

The issue is "How do we do it?"

If a healthcare organization had a financial problem, management would install a three-step process:

- Financial planning
- Financial controls
- Financial improvement

Management has formal financial goals, budgets, and review processes

Follow financial approach in managing for quality

Trilogy:

1. Quality planning
2. Quality goals
3. Quality improvement

Trilogy 1:
Quality Planning

Set business goals and develop means for meeting goals

■ Define quality from customer's view

■ Identify customers

■ Determine customer needs

■ Develop product/service features to meet needs

■ Establish product/service goals

■ Develop process to meet goals

■ Provide feedback

Poor planning is the source of poor quality

Planning improvements can occur only with feedback

Trilogy 2:
Quality Goals

Run the process that meets the product and service goals

Employees usually do **NOT** have the means for improvement

The best most employees can do is to meet what is planned in the process

Self-Control

Occurs when people have the means for:

■ Knowing their specific quality goals

■ Knowing their performance against goals

■ Correcting their performance if they are not meeting their goals

Trilogy 3:
Quality Improvement

Clear responsibility for improvement

■ Full top-management participation

■ **NOT** "here comes another drive" syndrome

Quality council with upper management membership

■ Develop process for selecting jobs for improvement

■ Provide review and recognition

■ Revise merit ratings for quality improvements

■ Business plan must include quality improvement goals

Role of facilitator:

■ Work with management to implement above

Juran's Audit

Break into your assigned teams.

Then select a healthcare organization, and using Juran's trilogy as a guide:

■ Identify three of their strongest points

■ Identify three of their weakest points

Why?

Be creative in your analysis.

Exercise 4: Your Analysis

Did:

- **YOU** try to change **YOUR** behavior?

- Each member contribute equally?

- Anyone dominate the discussion?

- Anyone not make a contribution?

- The leader call on specific members by name?

- Anyone practice positive reinforcement?
  Provide specific examples of the positive reinforcement used

For the next exercise:

- Practice positive reinforcement

- All team members should be equally prepared to give a report on the team's findings

- All members must be prepared to explain what they did differently to change **THEIR** behavior

JCAHO
Joint Commission on Accreditation for Health Care Organizations

Ten Steps of Monitoring and Evaluation

Step 1   Assign responsibility

Step 2   Delineate scope of care

Step 3   Identify important aspects of care

Step 4   Identify indicators

Step 5   Establish thresholds for evaluation

Step 6   Collect and organize data

Step 7   Evaluate care

Step 8   Take action to solve identified problems

Step 9   Assess action and document improvements

Step 10   Communicate relevant information to the quality assurance program

Chapter 3

Empowerment

Objective

To develop an understanding of what is expected of team members working in empowered teams

Pages

Pages 61–83 in *Healthcare Teams: Building Continuous Quality Improvement*

Exercises

5   What Is Empowerment?

6   Team Process Control

7   Measuring Medical Quality

Transparencies

3-1   Team Development

3-2   Student Advisors

3-3   Meaningful Quality

3-4   Changes Required for CQI

3-5   Empowered Firms

3-6   Team Empowerment: Team Responsibilities

3-7   Team Empowerment: Shared Responsibilities

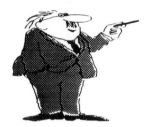

Exercise 6 (Team Process Control) can be a real eye-opener. Many participants want team empowerment because they feel the concept gives them more power, which it does. However, with the additional power comes responsibility for monitoring the process and taking corrective action immediately when needed. That is, the empowered team must assume responsibility for its portion of the process.

It might be a good idea to return to Exercise 7 (Measuring Medical Quality) and find out if the participants have additional factors to incorporate in the measurement.

Transparency 3-13 (Exercise: Your Analysis) asks team members what they did to change their team behavior. This can be used to prompt discussions.

Team Development

I. Traditional Hierarchy

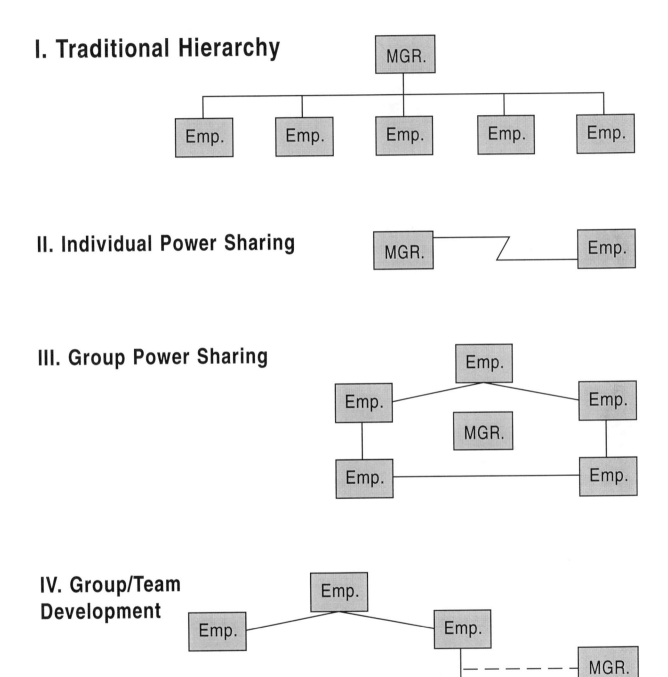

II. Individual Power Sharing

III. Group Power Sharing

IV. Group/Team Development

Student Advisors

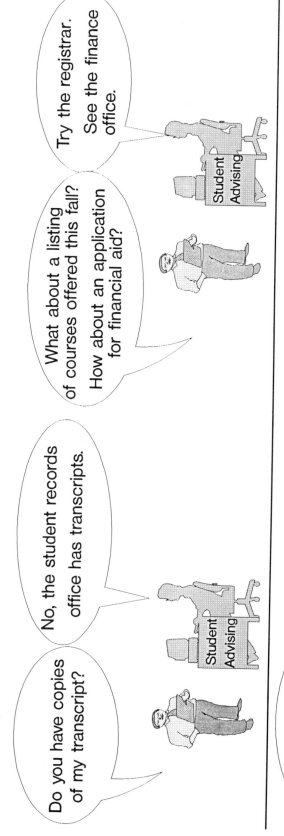

Do you have copies of my transcript?

No, the student records office has transcripts.

Student Advising

What about a listing of courses offered this fall? How about an application for financial aid?

Try the registrar. See the finance office.

Student Advising

How about a college catalog? A parking permit? A campus map?

Try the bookstore. See the public safety office. Try student affairs.

Student Advising

Thanks for your assistance.

Let me know if I can be of further help.

Student Advising

3-2

Meaningful Quality

For quality to be a personal and an organizational value, it must:

- Be chosen freely

- Be chosen from alternatives

- Be acted upon by the person and the organization

- Help people achieve their potential and help the organization achieve its potential

- Be publicly affirmed by the person and the organization

Changes Required for CQI

Issues	Change from:	Change to:
Defects	Inevitable	Zero defects
Training	Cost	Investment
Change	Resisted	Way of life
Time horizon	Short term	Long term
Customers	Take it or leave it	Satisfaction
Vendors	Price	Price and quality
Performance	Cost and schedule	Customer requirements
Information flow	Vertical	Horizontal and vertical
Performance goals	Standards	Better than yesterday
Management role	Enforcer	Coach

Empowered Firms

■ Accomplish work through independent teams

■ Foster an environment that develops, encourages, and rewards empowered people and teams

■ Encourage people to build social and technical skills

■ Align personal and organizational goals and see that people understand their roles

■ Exhibit a high level of individual and team self-management

■ Participate in work design, set direction, and resolve problems

■ Provide people with the information they need—without asking

Team Empowerment

Team responsibilities:

69%   Safety and housekeeping

58   Assign tasks to members

53   Work with internal customers

46   Stop work for quality issues

45   Routine equipment maintenance

44   Vacation scheduling

42   Process improvements

38   Select work methods

34   External customers

33   Determine training needs

29   Set production goals

Team Empowerment

Shared responsibilities:

54%   Select work methods

53   Determine training methods

51   Process improvements

49   Set production goals

54   Individual performance problems

44   Routine equipment maintenance

44   External customers

Supervisor responsibilities:

70%   Compensation decisions

55   Prepare and manage budgets

46   Performance appraisals

41   Individual performance problems

Team Empowerment:
Barriers to Success

■ Personnel issues

■ Supervisor resistance

■ Transfer of power to teams

■ Misalignment (compensation and team structure)

■ Difficulty with team members and supervisors in new roles

* See Kast and Laughlin, "Views on Self-Directed Workteams," *Journal for Quality and Participation,* pp. 48–51, Dec. 1990.

Self-Control

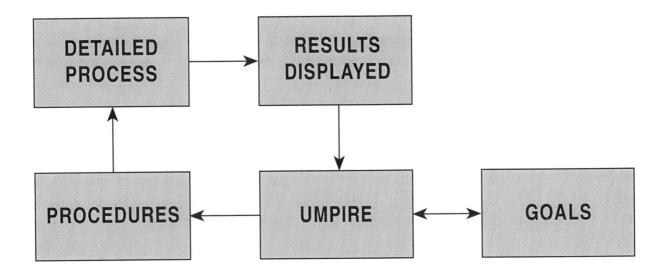

Umpire must have the means to control the process

Results must be easy to understand

Employees require:

Supportive environment

Open communication, free from fear

Data Processing Errors

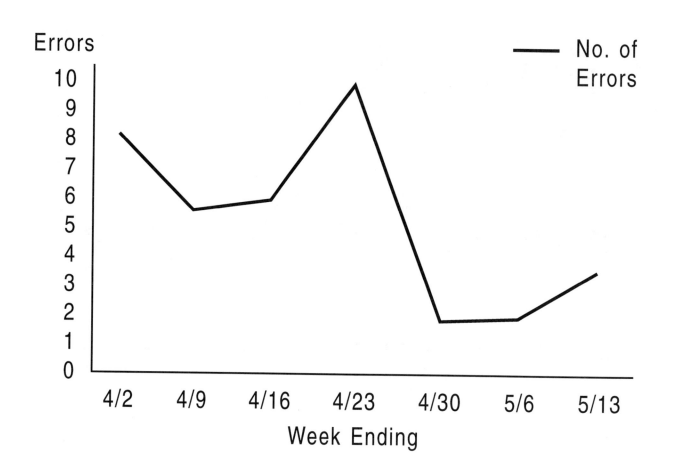

Errors

Documents Containing Incorrect Data

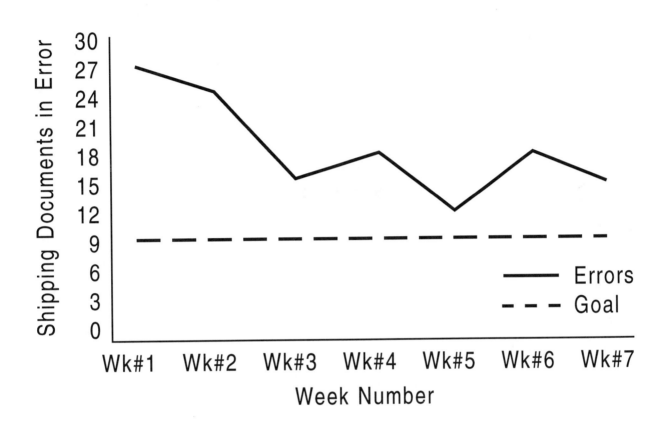

Empowerment: Application

Break into your assigned teams

Select a critical process

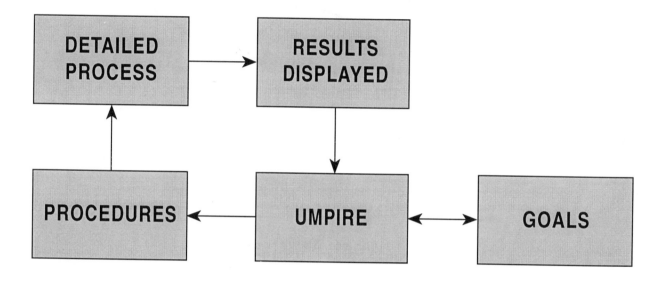

Design the specific results to be displayed

Exercise: Your Analysis

■ Was it awkward not knowing who would give the team's report?

■ If so, why was it awkward?

■ Provide specific examples of the positive reinforcement used

■ What did **YOU** do differently this time to change your behavior?

From now on:

■ Think in terms of how you moved the team forward

■ Always rotate all roles, including team leadership

It is the job of each team member to:

■ Be aware of the effect he or she has on the team

■ Move the conversation forward

■ Practice positive reinforcement when appropriate

Chapter 4

Supportive Team Cultures

Objective	To understand the characteristics of an effective team
Pages	Pages 85–96 in *Healthcare Teams: Building Continuous Quality Improvement*
Exercises	8 And In This Corner, Weighing 105 Pounds, We Have Nurse…
	9 Admissions Problem
Transparencies	4-1 Teams Need Creative and Empirical Thinkers
	4-2 Sample Team Rules (Part 1)
	4-3 Sample Team Rules (Part 2)

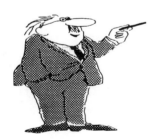

Follow through with the need for team members to fully understand that they have a responsibility to the team. Unproductive members should be ejected. It is better to do this in a learning environment than to suffer the harsh realities of a failure to perform in an organization.

Any team worth its salt could identify the classic problem in Exercise 8. A Registered Nurse (RN) has a two-year degree, while a Licensed Practical Nurse (LPN) has a one-year degree. (The four-year program is a bachelor's degree.) An LPN can do everything an RN can do, except start an IV. Frequently, an LPN receives about half the pay of an RN.

Teams Need
Creative and Empirical Thinkers

	Creative Thinking	Empirical Thinking

List Problems
Prioritize Problems

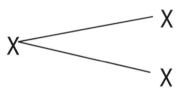

Analyze Symptoms
Formulate Theories
Test Theories

Identifying Root Causes

Consider Alternative Solutions
Design Solutions & Controls
Address Resistance
Implement Controls

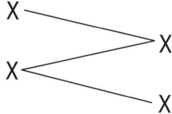

Implementing Solution

Check Performance   X
Monitor Control System   X

Sample Team Rules (Part 1)

- Regular meetings will be determined by team members.

- Four team members must be present for a meeting, which will constitute a quorum. The meeting will start and end on time, and members should be prepared to participate.

- If a member misses more than two unexcused team meetings, that member is dropped from the team.

- Members may be dropped from a team for failing to attend meetings or for failing to actively contribute to the team.

- A vote of 75% or more of the team is needed to drop a member from a team. (This 75% vote does not include the member to be removed.) The instructor/facilitator is to be notified of the name of the team member(s) who is no longer on the team and the reason he or she was removed from the team.

- Team members must be committed to attending all meetings. An effort should be made to accommodate the varying schedules of team members. However, if a member cannot attend due to work or any other reason, that member is not contributing to the team and will be dropped from the team.

Sample Team Rules (Part 2)

■ The last ten minutes of each meeting will be used to critique performance of team members and prepare the agenda for the next team meeting.

■ Service roles, including team leader, recorder, and observer, will be determined by team members. Assignment of these roles is to rotate and is to be determined at the end of each meeting.

■ The designated recorder will record minutes of the meeting and file them in a Master Minutes Book which will be maintained for the team. Also, the Observer's Recording Form (to be discussed) must be completed for each meeting and filed in the Master Minutes Book (held by a designated team member).

■ This minutes book must be turned in to the instructor/ facilitator when designated for review. In addition, the minutes book must accompany the final QI project.

■ Prior to turning in the minutes book, each team member is to anonymously complete a Peer Evaluation Form, which is turned in to the instructor/facilitator.

Chapter 5

Team-Building Phases

Objective	To be able to use performance feedback to improve individual and team effectiveness
Pages	Pages 97–116 in *Healthcare Teams: Building Continuous Quality Improvement*
Exercises	10 Written Team Rules
	11 Team Assessment
	12 General Peer Feedback
	13 Detailed Peer Evaluation
	14 Self-Assessment
Transparencies	5-1 Teams versus Groups
	5-2 Do's and Don'ts When Giving Feedback

Team   versus   Group

Team	Group
Decisions made by consensus with all inputs heard and valued	Groups tend to have majority and minority opinions
Disagreements are carefully examined and resolution is sought	Criticism tends to be destructive and disagreements are not effectively dealt with
Objectives are well understood and accepted by the team	Group members do not necessarily accept common objectives
Free expression of ideas occurs and others listen to what is said	Personal feelings are hidden
Self-examination of how the group is functioning frequently occurs	Discussions are avoided regarding how the group is functioning
Roles are understood by all members	Individuals tend to protect their role and their niche in the group
Shared leadership occurs on an as-needed basis	Leadership is appointed

A Few Do's and Don'ts When Giving Feedback

DO	DON'T
Be positive and thank members for the specific contributions they made.	Say "everyone did a good job." (Identify what each specific individual did or did not contribute.)
Be specific when someone's actions hurt the team. Try to provide positive feedback: "I understand your strong feelings regarding the proposal, but we needed to reach a group consensus we all could live with."	Say "your constant complaining annoyed me." (Phrase the sentence objectively and provide a specific example.)
Be clear. For example, if the issue was a failure to offer useful team input, state: "If you would have expressed your ideas on developing team rules more positively, I'm sure the group would have been more willing to include your suggestions."	Get involved in trivia such as, "Your failure to make eye contact decreases your effectiveness."

Chapter 6

Understanding How We Think

Objective	To understand the importance of trust, and to understand how we think
Pages	Pages 117–126 in *Healthcare Teams: Building Continuous Quality Improvement*
Exercises	15 Norm Violation
	16 Pardon Me, Doctor, But…
	17 The Room Is Not Clean?
Transparency	6-1 Hat Colors and Functions

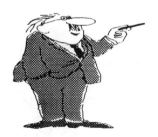

Exercise 16 (Pardon Me, Doctor, But…) is designed to identify the systems that are, or should be, in place at your medical facility and to encourage input into and discussion of items concerning the health and safety of the patient. Do the nurses have meaningful input into the doctors' decisions, and are they really encouraged to voice their opinions? Many medical centers often operate under a "fear syndrome," which minimizes meaningful input from key people in the system.

Hat Colors and Functions

White Hat
Mr. Clean

White is neutral and objective. The white hat is concerned with objective facts and figures.

Red Hat
The Alarmist

Red suggests alarm, anger (seeing red), rage, and emotion. The red hat gives the emotional view.

Purple Hat
The Pessimist

Purple covers the gloomy and negative aspects. The hat reflects why something cannot be done.

Yellow Hat
Susie Sunshine

Yellow is sunny, positive, and optimistic. It indicates new ideas, creativity, and moving forward.

Blue Hat
Cool Hand Luke

Blue is cool. Blue suggests control and organization of the thinking process. The blue hat defines the problem and summarizes the contributions of others.

Chapter 7

Member Service Roles

Objective	To identify the multiple service roles that must be performed if a team is to be effective
Pages	Pages 127–136 in *Healthcare Teams: Building Continuous Quality Improvement*
Exercises	18 Declining Patients
	19 Why Can't You Return My Phone Calls?
	20 My Son, The Future Doctor
Transparency	7-1 Observer's Recording Form

Observer's Recording Form: Participant Interactions

	Participant Names										
Hat Colors White											
Red											
Purple											
Yellow											
Blue											

Date:

Comments:

Observer:

Team #:

Assignment:

Chapter 8

Expanded Team Member Roles

Objective

To introduce member service roles, and to stress the observer's role so that teams can improve their performance

Pages

Pages 137–156 in *Healthcare Teams: Building Continuous Quality Improvement*

Exercises

21 Please Answer the Phone

22 No, We Can't Improve Our Medical Services

23 Pill Pusher Blues

24 Maintenance, When?

Transparencies

8-1 Team Member Service Roles

8-2 Participant Responsibilities

8-3 Leader Responsibilities

8-4 Recorder and Observer Responsibilities

8-5 When You Observe

8-6 Timekeeper Responsibilities

8-7 Task Functions–Task Description

8-8 Task Observation Form

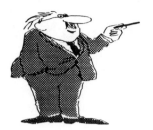

Exercise 21 (Please Answer the Phone) deals with the number one source of complaints, according to Ms. Beverly Nettles, Patient Advocate at the University of Louisville Medical Center, Louisville, Kentucky.

Team Member Service Roles

Participant   Actively discusses ideas and helps carry out what should be done

Leader   Guides the group as a coordinator/ facilitator

Recorder   Records pertinent ideas expressed and summarizes results at the end of each meeting

Observer   Observes the teamwork processes and discusses these observations at the end of each meeting

Resource Person   Used when needed on a planned discussion and addresses specific needs (not a speech)

Timekeeper   Watches the clock, schedules meetings, and reports on how the team productively utilizes its time

Trainer   Utilizes intervention to assist the team in learning how to learn

Participant responsibilities include:

- Being prepared

- Actively sharing ideas, without dominating the discussion

- Listening carefully

- Sharing ideas, experience, and expertise

- Building on others' contributions

- Helping with group functions: serving as leader, recorder, etc.

- Being flexible in terms of schedules, including meeting times

Leader responsibilities include:

- Making pre-meeting preparations

- Finalizing and distributing the agenda

- Helping establish, and then abiding by, team ground rules

- Keeping facilitator (in this case, the instructor) informed of progress

- Moving the group to a quality outcome by:

  - Shared planning

  - Shared appraisal

  - Free, voluntary expression

  - Acceptance of members as valuable individuals

Recorder responsibilities include:

- Reporting the essence of what was said about each topic (do not try to report every point)

- Recording the point that was made, **not** who said something

- Recording points on which opinions differ

- Recording points of agreement and decisions made

Observer responsibilities include:

- Providing a report on the group processes that occurred

- Being objective and limiting the report to what occurred, without inferring what should have been done

- Sitting so that he or she is facing the group and can see all members

- Making reference to the content of the discussion, but **not** keeping a running record of what was said

When you observe, consider the following teamwork process factors:

- Spontaneity of participation

- Balanced participation

- Emotional atmosphere

- Dependence on the discussion leader

- Helping others communicate

- Clarity of tasks and goals

- Building upon each other's contributions

- Quality of listening

- Factors that blocked progress toward the goal

Timekeeper responsibilities include:

- Watching the clock

- Setting a time limit for the meeting

- Reminding others of time remaining

- Reporting time usage

- Attending meeting with a calendar to facilitate scheduling the next meeting

Task Functions	Task Description
Initiating	Proposing tasks, defining problems, coordinating, clarifying, or suggesting an idea
Giving Information	Providing facts or information to assist the team in making a decision
Energizing	Motivating the team to make a greater effort
Evaluating or Criticizing	Judging the evidence and conclusions the team suggests

Task Observation Form

Tasks		Participant Names										
	Initiating											
	Giving Information											
	Energizing											
	Evaluating/ Criticizing											

Date: Observer:

Chapter 9

Expanding Team Skills

Objective	To practice learning how to improve our team performance
Pages	Pages 157–180 in *Healthcare Teams: Building Continuous Quality Improvement*
Exercises	25 Nurse, I'm Hungry
	26 Staff Problems
	27 Where Do I Park?
	28 Insurance Hassles
	29 Now What?
	30 Team Assessment
Transparencies	9-1 Phases of a Meeting (Part 1)
	9-2 Phases of a Meeting (Part 2)
	9-3 Communication Process
	9-4 Constructive Feedback Guidelines
	9-5 Solving Common Team Problems
	9-6 What Can Be Done to Overcome These Blocks?
	9-7 Exercise 29: Now What?

Phases of a Meeting (Part 1)

Before the Meeting

Leader	Participant
Establish meeting date and time	Confirm attendance
Secure a meeting room	Be flexible regarding when you can meet
Define objectives of meeting in an agenda	Define your role at the meeting
Notify participants	Do any required homework

During the Meeting

Leader	Participant
Start on time	Arrive on time
Follow the agenda	Actively contribute to the discussion
Elicit balanced participation	Limit side conversations and distractions
Help resolve conflicts	Be open-minded to ideas
Clarify action to be taken	Listen to and respect the opinions of others
Try to achieve consensus, and do not resort to voting	Participate in consensus with an open mind

Phases of a Meeting (Part 2)

After the Meeting, but Before Team Leaves

Leader	Participant
Ensure time for observer's report	Reflect on your actions
Summarize results	Give up personal ownership to team ownership
Ensure that roles are rotated and that participants accept new roles	Ask yourself what you have learned regarding group interactions
Introduce new leader and new observer	

After the Meeting and the Team Has Left

Leader	Participant
Reflect on balanced contribution, and if you were able to stay out of discussions	Take any action agreed to
Restore room and return equipment	Follow up on action items
Ensure that the recorder distributes meeting notes	Think about what you should do differently during the next team meeting

Communication Process

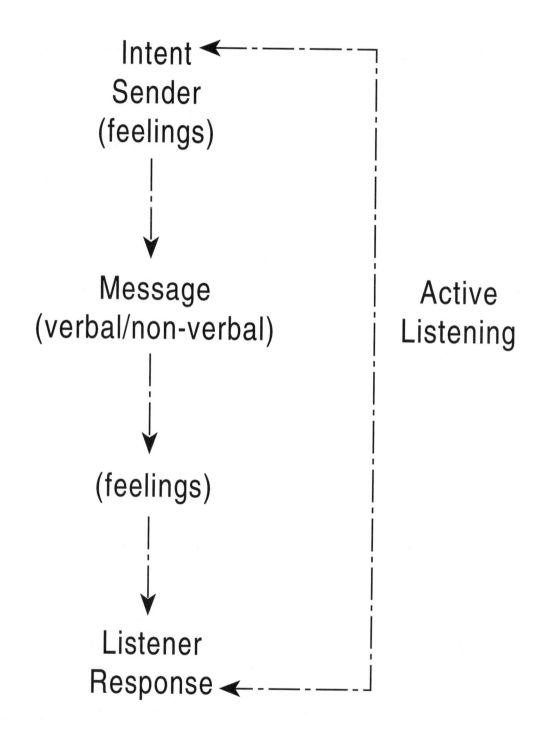

Intent
Sender
(feelings)

Message
(verbal/non-verbal)

(feelings)

Listener
Response

Active
Listening

No one willingly communicates badly.

Constructive Feedback Guidelines

■ **Give positive and negative feedback**

■ **Understand the context**

■ **Know how to give feedback**

    ■ Be descriptive

    ■ Don't exaggerate

    ■ Speak for yourself

■ **Know how to receive feedback**

    ■ Listen carefully

    ■ Ask questions for clarity

    ■ Acknowledge valid points

    ■ Carefully consider the points

    ■ Don't get angry

How Would You Recommend We Solve These Common Team Problems?

- Talkative team member

- Dominant team member

- Reluctant participant

- Argumentative team members

- Lack of team focus

What can be done
to overcome these blocks?

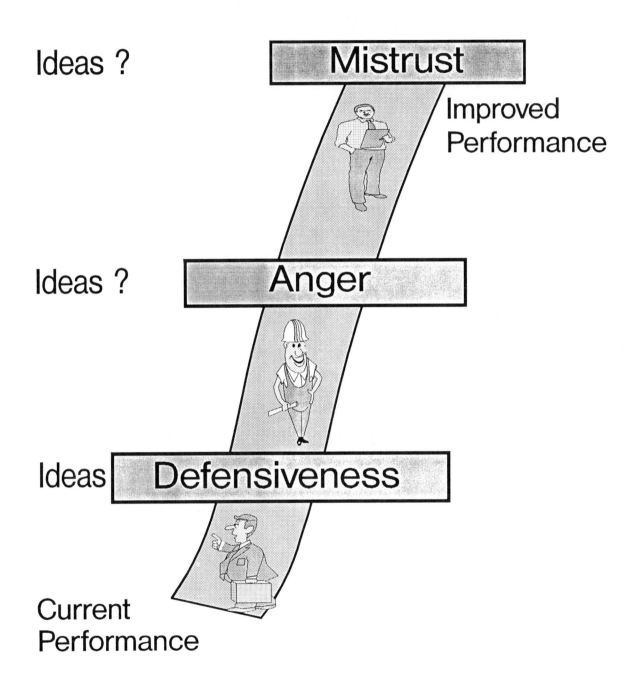

Ideas ?
Mistrust

Improved
Performance

Ideas ?
Anger

Ideas Defensiveness

Current
Performance

Exercise 29: Now What?

- Your first choice should be the mirror, because it makes an excellent long-distance signaling device. Although you are alone, you are likely to see vehicles or planes in the distance.

- The hat is a likely second choice, because shade will definitely be a problem.

- Although the ax is important, its weight will be a hindrance on a long hike.

- The salt tablets are virtually worthless. Numerous other problems will occur before you have to worry about a salt deficiency.

- Matches are your first choice, for starting a fire to overcome the cold nights.

- The baseball bat is your second choice. It might make you feel more secure.

- The high proof of the alcohol will speed up dehydration and hasten your death. Although the high proof could be handy in starting a fire, most things you find in the desert will already be dry. Get rid of the alcohol.

- Drink as much as you need to avoid dehydration. Once dehydration starts, your limited water will do little to stop the process.

- Your first choice should be to ask the genie to transport you to the nearest city.

- Don't push your luck by telling him to go away.

- $5 million in gold weighs 1000 pounds, which would flatten your greedy little body.

Chapter 10

Teams, Teams, and More Teams

Objective	To become familiar with specialized types of teams
Pages	Pages 181–192 in *Healthcare Teams: Building Continuous Quality Improvement*
Exercises	None
Transparencies	10-1 Quality Teams
	10-2 What Is the Function of the Following Types of Teams?
	10-3 Steps in Developing Design Teams
	10-4 Quality Council
	10-5* Quality Council: Need
	10-6* Quality Council: Employee's Role

* These topics are not in the book. They may be used to expand the discussion if desired.

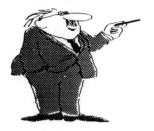

Note the additional quality council transparency masters denoted by an asterisk (*). Have these available to explore the concepts in greater depth, if desired.

Quality, like the weather, is a topic everyone talks about. Without the focus of a quality council, there will be no systematic way to follow through on quality improvement ideas.

Quality Teams

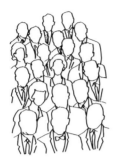
Customers

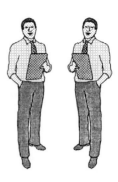
Employees

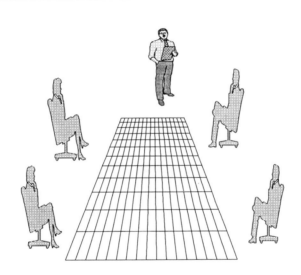

Quality Teams

What Is the Function of the Following Types of Teams?

- Task teams

- Project teams

- Functional teams

- Self-directed teams

- Design teams

Steps in Developing Design Teams

- Organization is committed to finding a better way

- Quality council/teams investigate what others are doing

- Executive group clarifies the mission

- Quality council appoints a design team

- Read about similar groups and visit sites

- Analyze environment, technology, and jobs

- Discuss draft plan with involved groups

- Make recommendations to quality council

- Implement design and evaluate

Quality Council

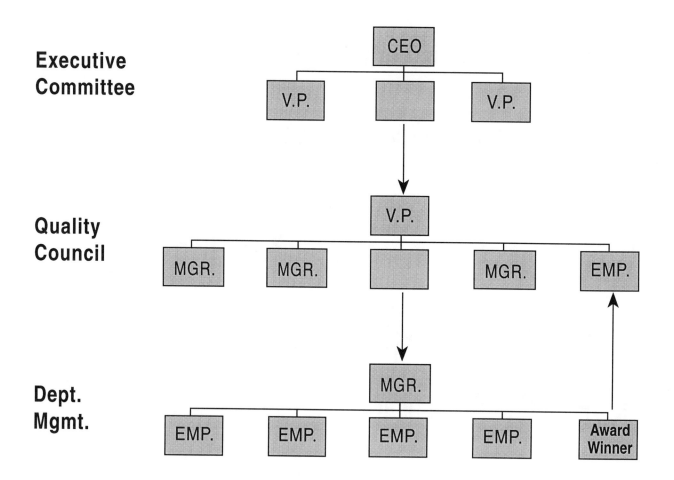

Executive Committee

Quality Council

Dept. Mgmt.

Quality Council: Need

There is no problem in identifying improvement ideas

■ Your employees have hundreds of excellent ideas

■ Follow-through is needed!

Quality ideas are discussed, then put on the back burner because:

■ Problems are not placed on an authoritative agenda

■ There was no clear responsibility assigned to solve the problem

■ No one realized that a team was required

A structure is needed to choose projects, assign responsibility, and follow up on implementation

Quality Council: Employee's Role

Phases I and II:

- Read about successful quality projects

- Discuss quality articles circulated

Phase III:

- Discuss successful CQI projects in department meetings with award winners

Phase IV:

- Evaluations stress CQI participation

- Opportunity for Improvement Program (ideas are part of every job)

- Participate in quality projects

- Letters of recommendation

- Attendance at quality seminars

- CQI savings

- Other quality contributions

Appendix A

Quality Bucks

The forms in this section are presented in a format that facilitates photocopying. The quality bucks are very attractive if copied on green paper. It is relatively easy to run the front of the 50, 100, and 200 quality bucks through a copier. Then trim them close to the border, and you are off and running. The appendix contains:

Front   **Back**

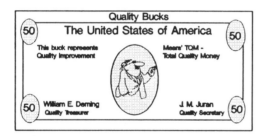
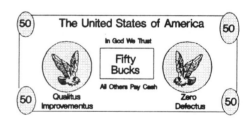

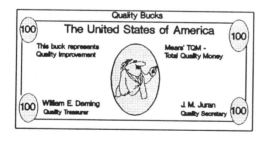
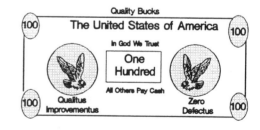

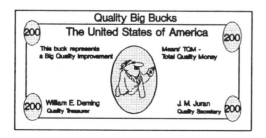
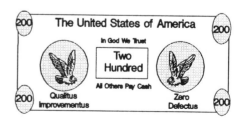

You will need a lot of these quality bucks, because people tend to eagerly want them. Hence they are arranged three-up to conserve paper when photocopying. You will find that all age groups appreciate receiving the bucks—but be stingy with them. Don't reward poor ideas, and make people earn the 200 denomination bucks by awarding them only for innovative quality ideas.

These bucks are proof to the participants that their quality ideas make a difference. If time permits, and if you have some inexpensive memorabilia available, then have a quality auction at the end of the sessions. This auction will serve two purposes. First, it will reward the innovators. Second, it will also reward those people who have learned to operate together in a team and therefore pooled their bucks to obtain the prizes.

If you want to get fancy, and if you have access to a double-sided copier, copy the front and back of a denomination on opposite sides of a single sheet of paper. Try a sample, because positioning of the masters on the copier will undoubtedly need to be adjusted. After copying the front and back, hold the copy made up to the light to see if the registration is acceptable. Then trim the front.

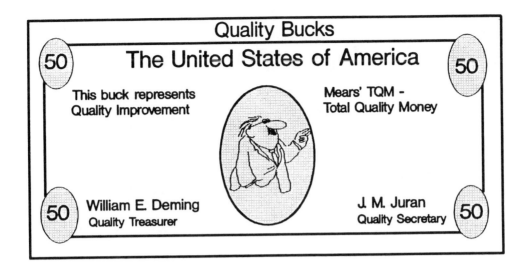

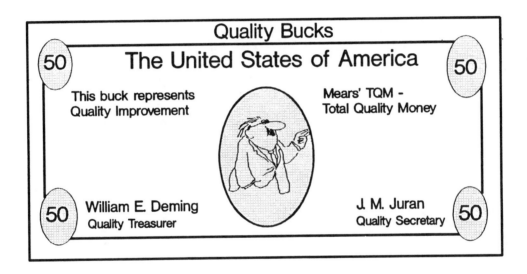

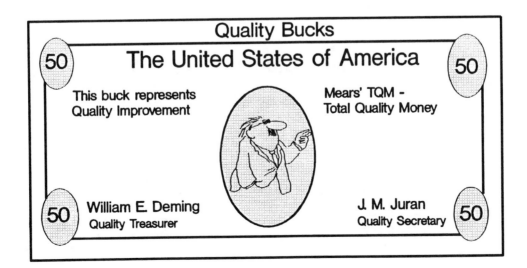

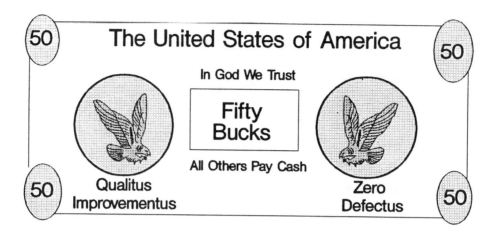

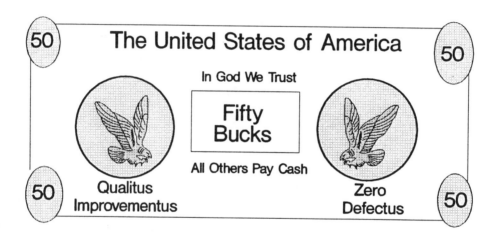

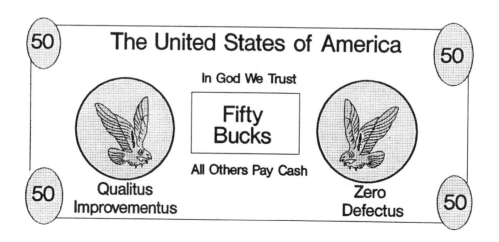

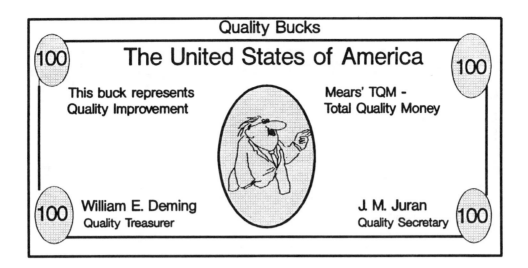

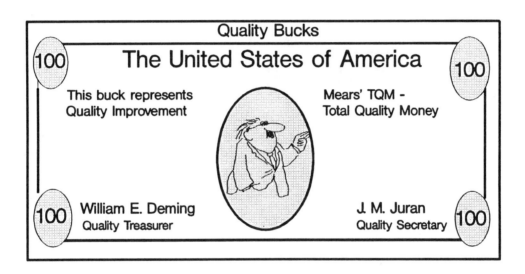

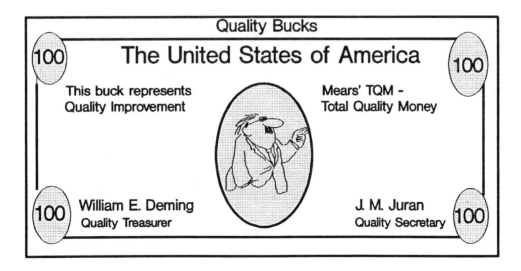

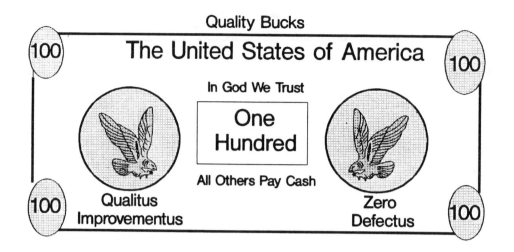

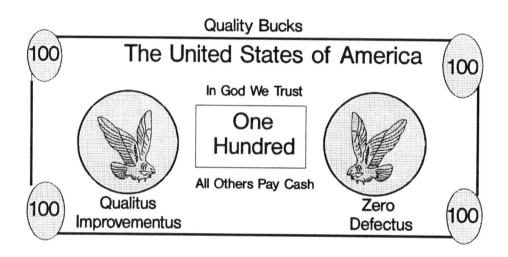

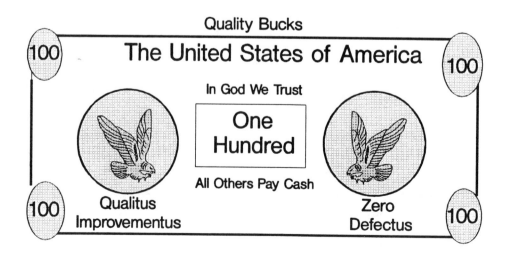

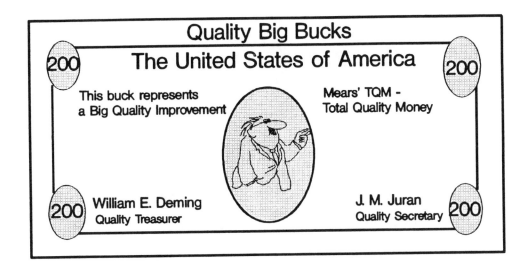

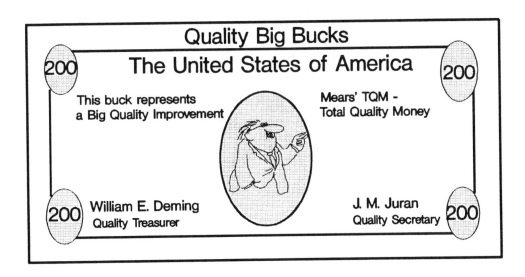

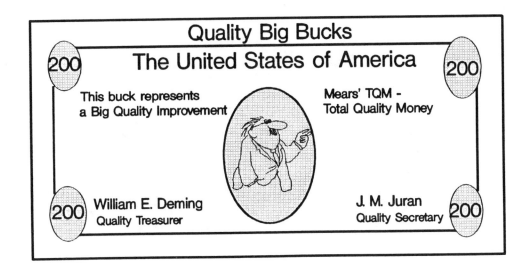

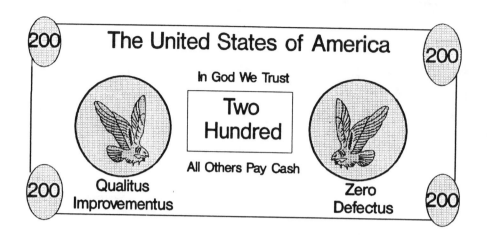

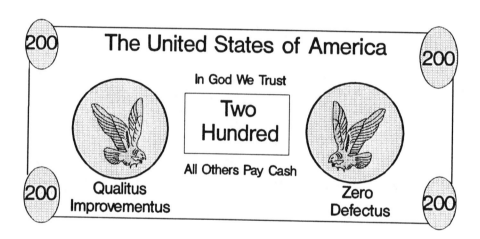

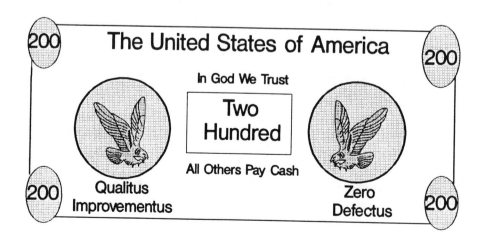

Appendix B

Random Team Assignments

This section presents a method for randomly assigning participants to teams. This technique is useful in order to give the participants experience in reaching consensus with varying team members.

Random team assignment tables are provided for up to five random team assignments with varying numbers of teams and participants. The process of using the random team assignment tables to assign participants to teams is as follows:

■ Record participant names on the form labeled Random Team Assignment Log. Two copies of this form are provided for your convenience.

■ Locate the random team assignment table for the number of participants in your session. If you can't find the exact number, use a table with fewer participants, and place the "overage" wherever you want.

For example, suppose you want to randomly assign the following nine participants to two teams:

1 Mary Worth	6 Richard Herden
2 John Smith	7 Bruce Kemelgor
3 Susie Sunshine	8 Lou Raho
4 Tom Jones	9 Dennis Buda
5 Alice James	

The random numbers for assigning nine participants to two teams are as follows for the first time the group is assigned:

Assignment: 1	Participant #/Team				
Team 1:	6	5	9	4	2
Team 2:	1	3	7	8	

Thus, team 1 contains the 6th participant, Richard Herden, as well as the 5th participant, Alice James. The complete membership of team 1 is Richard Herden, Alice James, Dennis Buda, Tom Jones, and John Smith. The remainder of the participants are assigned to team 2.

The most tedious part of the random assignment process is writing the participant names in the Random Team Assignment Log. If the names are recorded in a listing (gradebook, listing of participants, etc.), simply consecutively number the names and assign the appropriate team numbers.

The ideal team size is from five to six participants. The following random assignments begin with assigning eight participants to two teams, which at four people per team is a little under the ideal size for evaluating group interaction.

Random Team Assignment Log

Participant Number	Participant Name	Random Team Assignment
1		
2		
3		
4		
5		
6		
7		
8		
9		
10		
11		
12		
13		
14		
15		
16		
17		
18		
19		
20		
21		
22		
23		
24		
25		

Random Team Assignment Log		
Participant Number	**Participant Name**	**Random Team Assignment**
1		
2		
3		
4		
5		
6		
7		
8		
9		
10		
11		
12		
13		
14		
15		
16		
17		
18		
19		
20		
21		
22		
23		
24		
25		

Random Team Assignments: 8 participants to 2 teams

Assignment: 1   **Participant#/Team**
Team 1:   6   7   5   2
Team 2:   3   1   8   4

Assignment: 2   **Participant#/Team**
Team 1:   5   3   2   6
Team 2:   4   8   7   1

Assignment: 3   **Participant#/Team**
Team 1:   5   8   3   7
Team 2:   2   6   4   1

Assignment: 4   **Participant#/Team**
Team 1:   3   7   1   5
Team 2:   6   4   2   8

Assignment: 5   **Participant#/Team**
Team 1:   7   2   6   5
Team 2:   4   3   8   1

Random Team Assignments: 9 participants to 2 teams

Assignment: 1   **Participant #/Team**
Team 1:   6   5   9   4   2
Team 2:   1   3   7   8

Assignment: 2   **Participant #/Team**
Team 1:   2   8   6   4   9
Team 2:   1   5   3   7

Assignment: 3   **Participant #/Team**
Team 1:   1   5   2   3   4
Team 2:   7   8   6   9

Assignment: 4   **Participant #/Team**
Team 1:   7   6   1   8   5
Team 2:   9   4   2   3

Assignment: 5   **Participant #/Team**
Team 1:   6   2   1   8   9
Team 2:   5   3   7   4

Random Team Assignments: 10 participants to 2 teams

Assignment: 1   Participant #/Team

Team 1:	2	7	4	1	8
Team 2:	9	3	5	6	10

Assignment: 2   Participant #/Team

Team 1:	4	6	9	5	7
Team 2:	8	2	3	10	1

Assignment: 3   Participant #/Team

Team 1:	6	2	9	4	1
Team 2:	10	3	7	8	5

Assignment: 4   Participant #/Team

Team 1:	1	9	7	2	6
Team 2:	4	8	3	5	10

Assignment: 5   Participant #/Team

Team 1:	8	2	3	9	1
Team 2:	5	7	4	6	10

Random Team Assignments: 11 participants to 2 teams

Assignment: 1   Participant #/Team

Team 1:	10	1	11	6	3	8
Team 2:	9	5	7	4	2	

Assignment: 2   Participant #/Team

Team 1:	3	8	9	5	7	11
Team 2:	6	10	4	2	1	

Assignment: 3   Participant #/Team

Team 1:	5	10	7	6	8	4
Team 2:	2	3	9	1	11	

Assignment: 4   Participant #/Team

Team 1:	3	4	8	10	9	11
Team 2:	7	5	1	6	2	

Assignment: 5   Participant #/Team

Team 1:	5	8	7	9	6	11
Team 2:	2	1	10	4	3	

Random Team Assignments: 14 participants to 2 teams

Assignment: 1 Participant #/Team
Team 1: 3 10 4 6 1 2 11
Team 2: 13 5 8 9 12 7 14

Assignment: 2 Participant #/Team
Team 1: 12 7 1 8 4 5 13
Team 2: 3 10 9 2 11 6 14

Assignment: 3 Participant #/Team
Team 1: 3 11 8 12 4 5 7
Team 2: 6 2 9 10 13 1 14

Assignment: 4 Participant #/Team
Team 1: 12 8 10 1 5 2 13
Team 2: 6 4 7 11 9 3 14

Assignment: 5 Participant #/Team
Team 1: 12 3 13 10 11 14 6
Team 2: 9 2 7 4 1 5 8

Random Team Assignments: 14 participants to 3 teams

Assignment: 1 Participant #/Team
Team 1: 8 2 6 4 10
Team 2: 3 1 11 9 14
Team 3: 13 7 5 12

Assignment: 2 Participant #/Team
Team 1: 7 6 3 8 5
Team 2: 11 9 12 10 14
Team 3: 1 13 2 4

Assignment: 3 Participant #/Team
Team 1: 6 2 12 7 14
Team 2: 5 11 10 8 1
Team 3: 4 9 13 3

Assignment: 4 Participant #/Team
Team 1: 1 2 8 12 9
Team 2: 6 10 7 5 14
Team 3: 3 11 4 13

Assignment: 5 Participant #/Team
Team 1: 5 10 13 3 7
Team 2: 4 1 14 2 12
Team 3: 11 8 6 9

Random Team Assignments: 15 participants to 3 teams

Assignment: 1	Participant #/Team			
Team 1:	14	1	7	11	3
Team 2:	15	12	10	2	13
Team 3:	6	4	5	9	8

Assignment: 2	Participant #/Team			
Team 1:	7	2	14	6	3
Team 2:	11	9	4	10	8
Team 3:	5	13	12	15	1

Assignment: 3	Participant #/Team			
Team 1:	1	4	3	9	13
Team 2:	11	6	14	12	8
Team 3:	5	2	10	7	15

Assignment: 4	Participant #/Team			
Team 1:	13	14	11	9	3
Team 2:	1	4	7	2	12
Team 3:	15	8	6	5	10

Assignment: 5	Participant #/Team			
Team 1:	11	13	4	8	9
Team 2:	14	7	2	10	6
Team 3:	1	3	5	12	15

Random Team Assignments: 19 participants to 3 teams

Assignment: 1	Participant #/Team						
Team 1:	11	1	18	12	2	8	13
Team 2:	17	7	16	4	6	10	
Team 3:	9	5	14	3	15	19	

Assignment: 2	Participant #/Team						
Team 1:	5	3	9	13	6	14	4
Team 2:	8	19	10	16	11	12	
Team 3:	7	15	18	1	17	2	

Assignment: 3	Participant #/Team						
Team 1:	12	2	11	16	15	9	1
Team 2:	6	17	14	10	3	13	
Team 3:	19	7	8	4	5	18	

Assignment: 4	Participant #/Team						
Team 1:	4	6	14	3	9	11	17
Team 2:	5	7	16	13	12	1	
Team 3:	8	2	18	10	19	15	

Assignment: 5	Participant #/Team						
Team 1:	3	16	6	11	18	8	19
Team 2:	7	15	13	10	5	4	
Team 3:	17	2	9	1	12	14	

Random Team Assignments: 23 participants to 4 teams

Assignment: 1 Participant #/Team

Team 1:	6	11	8	18	10	5
Team 2:	2	21	14	12	4	22
Team 3:	3	19	20	1	15	23
Team 4:	9	13	7	17	16	

Assignment: 2 Participant #/Team

Team 1:	13	16	4	22	14	23
Team 2:	12	15	21	19	7	5
Team 3:	11	9	8	6	2	18
Team 4:	3	17	1	20	10	

Assignment: 3 Participant #/Team

Team 1:	11	3	9	14	10	21
Team 2:	4	13	18	5	7	6
Team 3:	8	1	15	23	17	22
Team 4:	20	16	12	19	2	

Assignment: 4 Participant #/Team

Team 1:	20	13	8	21	16	17
Team 2:	11	19	5	12	22	1
Team 3:	15	3	10	6	4	23
Team 4:	18	2	9	14	7	

Assignment: 5 Participant #/Team

Team 1:	7	16	14	1	20	23
Team 2:	19	15	2	17	11	10
Team 3:	21	22	4	8	3	13
Team 4:	5	6	12	9	18	

Random Team Assignments: 24 participants to 4 teams

Assignment: 1 **Participant #/Team**

Team 1:	7	10	9	18	14	1
Team 2:	24	15	20	4	3	17
Team 3:	6	21	11	16	22	12
Team 4:	13	23	2	8	19	5

Assignment: 2 **Participant #/Team**

Team 1:	24	21	5	3	22	23
Team 2:	19	14	10	15	16	4
Team 3:	6	8	17	13	2	18
Team 4:	7	12	11	1	9	20

Assignment: 3 **Participant #/Team**

Team 1:	15	23	21	9	10	4
Team 2:	7	14	11	17	2	13
Team 3:	18	8	19	6	20	3
Team 4:	5	22	12	16	24	1

Assignment: 4 **Participant #/Team**

Team 1:	7	5	4	16	14	8
Team 2:	18	2	21	23	17	19
Team 3:	15	3	10	9	12	11
Team 4:	6	13	20	24	22	1

Assignment: 5 **Participant #/Team**

Team 1:	4	24	1	12	6	11
Team 2:	18	13	19	5	16	15
Team 3:	2	14	22	7	3	8
Team 4:	21	9	10	20	23	17

Random Team Assignments: 25 participants to 5 teams

Assignment: 1 Participant #/Team

Team					
Team 1:	15	2	13	6	12
Team 2:	5	1	3	23	19
Team 3:	8	10	20	21	9
Team 4:	14	11	16	17	25
Team 5:	4	7	24	22	18

Assignment: 2 Participant #/Team

Team					
Team 1:	18	2	17	19	14
Team 2:	24	22	8	3	21
Team 3:	1	4	10	23	5
Team 4:	25	11	12	15	7
Team 5:	20	13	9	16	6

Assignment: 3 Participant #/Team

Team					
Team 1:	7	6	10	12	14
Team 2:	15	24	23	17	22
Team 3:	9	2	8	18	21
Team 4:	3	19	1	5	4
Team 5:	20	16	25	13	11

Assignment: 4 Participant #/Team

Team					
Team 1:	22	16	2	6	24
Team 2:	19	11	20	7	4
Team 3:	1	8	10	13	12
Team 4:	17	23	14	15	3
Team 5:	5	21	18	9	25

Assignment: 5 Participant #/Team

Team					
Team 1:	24	6	16	3	4
Team 2:	15	8	23	5	14
Team 3:	12	19	22	7	9
Team 4:	13	20	17	10	21
Team 5:	25	18	2	11	1

Random Team Assignments: 30 participants to 6 teams

Assignment: 1	Participant #/Team				
Team 1:	29	24	23	26	4
Team 2:	19	14	11	9	18
Team 3:	1	15	6	17	2
Team 4:	16	27	5	7	30
Team 5:	25	20	22	28	13
Team 6:	3	10	8	12	21

Assignment: 2	Participant #/Team				
Team 1:	29	25	27	24	26
Team 2:	2	3	14	10	9
Team 3:	28	16	23	5	15
Team 4:	12	13	4	8	1
Team 5:	11	18	21	7	20
Team 6:	6	19	22	30	17

Assignment: 3	Participant #/Team				
Team 1:	15	5	24	13	18
Team 2:	7	14	22	3	29
Team 3:	2	19	21	1	8
Team 4:	11	27	23	28	12
Team 5:	17	20	25	30	16
Team 6:	9	10	6	4	26

Assignment: 4	Participant #/Team				
Team 1:	26	18	3	22	17
Team 2:	7	28	30	15	4
Team 3:	24	10	2	12	11
Team 4:	6	23	29	20	25
Team 5:	27	19	21	9	13
Team 6:	5	8	14	16	1

Assignment: 5	Participant #/Team				
Team 1:	16	17	15	18	20
Team 2:	21	23	25	1	28
Team 3:	27	10	22	6	8
Team 4:	7	29	26	4	3
Team 5:	2	24	9	19	14
Team 6:	11	12	5	13	30

Random Team Assignments: 35 participants to 6 teams

Assignment: 1   Participant #/Team

Team						
Team 1:	17	30	21	10	8	27
Team 2:	18	12	6	24	4	15
Team 3:	32	22	31	20	28	35
Team 4:	9	25	23	34	2	3
Team 5:	7	33	5	13	14	29
Team 6:	19	1	11	16	26	

Assignment: 2   Participant #/Team

Team						
Team 1:	11	23	21	35	17	6
Team 2:	9	13	27	28	31	20
Team 3:	5	30	18	7	29	34
Team 4:	10	14	2	8	33	25
Team 5:	16	15	3	24	22	19
Team 6:	26	32	4	12	1	

Assignment: 3   Participant #/Team

Team						
Team 1:	17	20	26	25	21	22
Team 2:	3	28	27	31	13	9
Team 3:	10	5	24	8	32	35
Team 4:	1	7	18	4	34	12
Team 5:	15	16	33	29	19	11
Team 6:	14	30	6	23	2	

Assignment: 4   Participant #/Team

Team						
Team 1:	13	27	14	16	11	35
Team 2:	18	28	22	12	31	23
Team 3:	34	3	24	7	26	20
Team 4:	10	15	19	32	33	30
Team 5:	2	29	1	5	9	21
Team 6:	6	17	25	4	8	

Assignment: 5   Participant #/Team

Team						
Team 1:	35	5	34	33	27	25
Team 2:	14	31	23	15	9	28
Team 3:	18	6	3	7	1	19
Team 4:	32	11	10	17	13	12
Team 5:	2	16	30	24	26	4
Team 6:	8	22	29	21	20	

Appendix C

Hats Off Award

The purpose of studying and practicing team-building concepts is to learn how to work together in a team. The Hats Off Award is a way for the instructor/facilitator to say "thanks" to those who have tried extra hard to make a contribution to their team.

Participants are recognized for their contributions through an award given at the end of the course. However, no awards may be given if the general level of participation and learning is not sufficient to warrant recognition.

Two awards may be given to each team based on:

■ **Peer Recognition:** Team participants will be asked to select one of their own for the award. The person selected could be the one who contributed the most to improve the learning performance of the team.

■ **Instructor Recognition:** A trainee will be selected based on who has grown the most as a learner and who has demonstrated such growth by assisting his or her team.

Remind participants that when they are reading the material and participating in the exercises, the important point is not what they memorized. The important point is for everyone to be willing to change his or her behavior to improve their effectiveness in teams.

Two Hats Off Award certificates are provided:

■ **Certificate of Quality Achievement:** When this team-building book is used as a portion of a quality improvement effort.

■ **Certificate of Achievement:** When this book is used as a "pure" team-building course.

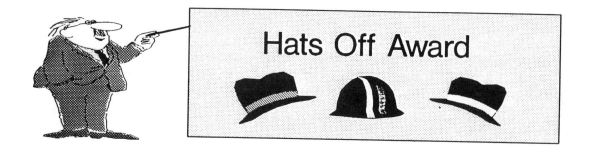

Hats Off Award

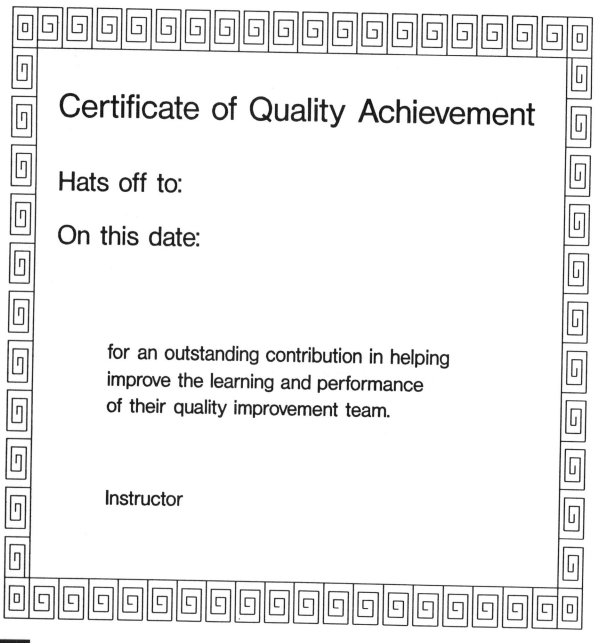

Certificate of Quality Achievement

Hats off to:

On this date:

for an outstanding contribution in helping
improve the learning and performance
of their quality improvement team.

Instructor

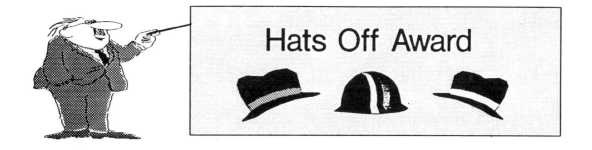

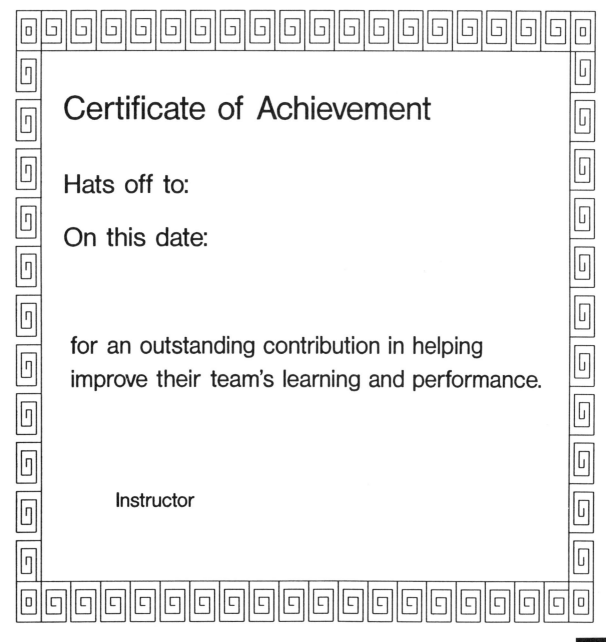

Certificate of Achievement

Hats off to:

On this date:

for an outstanding contribution in helping
improve their team's learning and performance.

Instructor

Appendix D

Team Presentations

I have teams "carry the ball" and present the results of their exercises to the class as a whole. This can be a positive learning experience, as the presentations expose participants to the wealth of different approaches that different teams develop.

On the negative side, frankly some presentations are boring. To develop excitement and to promote competition among teams, I suggest telling the group something on the order of the following:

> We are going to follow the olympic grading method for all presentations. Team presentations are graded on a score of one to ten for both technical content and artistic content. We are not going to "whack anyone on the knees" if a team doesn't do a good job in both categories, but quality bucks are awarded only for superior presentations.

An Olympic Scoring Form used for feedback to the groups is provided.

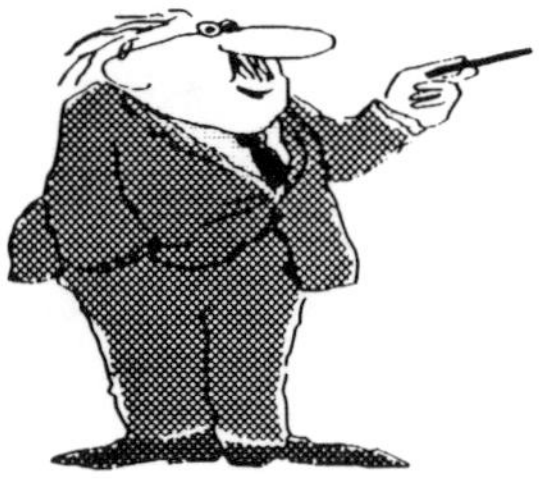

Team Presentations
Olympic Scoring Points

Scoring:

Technical ____________

Artistic ____________

Subtotal ____________

Deductions* ____________

Net Score ____________

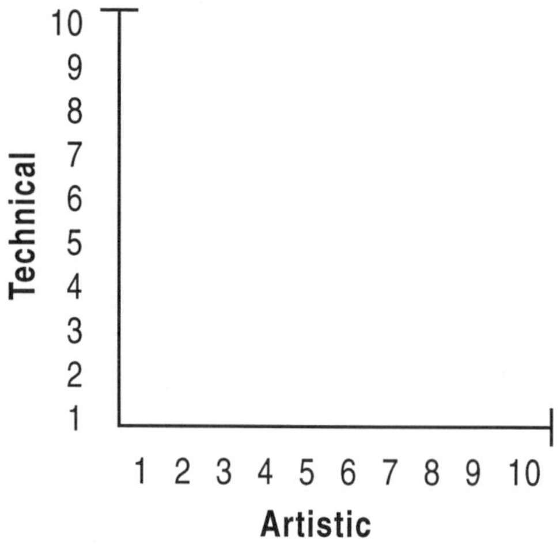
Technical
10
9
8
7
6
5
4
3
2
1
1 2 3 4 5 6 7 8 9 10
Artistic

* One point deducted for each person reading to group

A score above 9 is reserved for super-human effort

Comments/Suggestions for Improving:

Team # ____________ **Date** ____________

Instructor ________________________